AMAZING
BATH EXPERIENCE

~~~

By Emily Taylor
~~~

TABLE OF CONTENTS

Whip Up the Dream Bath You Deserve 5

Benefits You Gain from a Good Bath..6

The Essential Oils 9

Aromatherapy 16

All About Bath Soaps and Soap Making.. 19

Oils for Soap Making.. 21

Homemade Soap Recipes 25

Shampoos 35

Bath Bombs 44

Bath Salts 53

Body Scrubs 58

Body Lotion / Moisturizer... 63

Body Butters.. 70

Face Masks 73

WHIP UP THE DREAM BATH YOU DESERVE

One of the best feelings there is, especially after a long day at work, would be indulging in a relaxing bath. Even the ancients believed that cleanliness brings a person closer to the gods; and this must be the reason why until today, the adage that says cleanliness is next to godliness still rings true.

However, it sometimes happens that this fast-paced world deprives us of this luxury. We have to be mindful of our time and indulgences are often set aside. It could be that your day starts very early in the morning and your schedule only allow you a quick, often cold, morning shower. It could be that your workdays have you handcuffed to long working hours; leaving you a little too tired to prep for a soothing bath. Instead, you just opt for yet another quick shower before going to bed.

If such is your predicament, it is time for you to reserve at least 20 minutes of your time on weekends to treat yourself to a good long bath. A good bath does not simply mean unceremoniously immersing yourself in water. For it to work its magic, treat it more like a ritual.

A good bath is a purification rite. You put together special items and go through a checklist of procedures that you perform in an almost sacred manner. You get into a bath tired and weary; and come out of it completely rejuvenated and confident. As if the water has washed away any restlessness and healed your aching body.

And that feeling? It isn't just in your head. Science has proven that a good bath can also be very good for your health!

BENEFITS YOU GAIN FROM A GOOD BATH

• RIDS YOUR BODY OF TOXINS.

For effective detoxification, you need a tub of warm water with temps of about 90°F. At this temperature, your pores would open and allow sweating, consequently helping in the release of toxins. This is also the perfect temperature for relief from slight colds, and muscle and joint pains. A detoxifying bath also jumpstarts your digestive system to work properly providing you relief from constipation. Soak time is 10-20 minutes.

• IMPROVES CIRCULATION

A warm bath causes your veins and arteries to swell, encouraging better blood flow. This is particularly helpful in dealing with varicose veins and other circulatory problems. Soak time is 15 minutes.

• CURES COLDS AND HEADACHES

The scented steam emanating from your hot bath works wonders for clogged noses and persistent coughs. The steam helps loosen the mucus in your nose; and returns your breathing to normal. It also aids in flushing mucus buildup by moisturizing dry air passageways.

Add a few drops of essential oils such as lemon, lavender, thyme or peppermint in your warm bath. Soak time is 10 to 20 minutes. Finish off with a quick rinse of cold water.

• DE-STRESSES

If you're full of tension, a cold bath is the perfect way to de-stress. A cold bath means soaking in waters around 55-65°F. That's really cold and you have to be in tiptop shape to brave such low temperatures. Cold baths have the opposite effect of warm baths. A cold bath thins the blood resulting in increased blood sugar levels. Soak time is 30 seconds, tops.

• HELPS FIGHT INFECTION

Adding about four cups of organic cider vinegar to your warm bath is a good way to protect you from yeast infection. The cider vinegar also helps in detoxification and restoration of your body's acid-alkaline balance. Soak time should not exceed 20 minutes.

• HELPS CURE INSOMNIA

A cold bath brings amazing results if you have trouble sleeping. Soak for 20 minutes or for as long as you can bear the cold.

• LOWERS BLOOD SUGAR LEVEL

A warm bath helps dilate the blood vessels. An increase in blood flow enables the body to make maximum use of insulin, the hormone that converts glucose into energy. Soak time should not exceed 30 minutes.

• AIDS IN RELAXATION, MEDITATION, OR QUIET THINKING

A long bath is your perfect guilt-free excuse to be alone all by yourself for a little me-time. It's provides you with complete isolation and quiet after a chaotic day.

It is during this moment of comfort and easiness that your brain takes a break and just lets your subconscious sort through all the clutter in your mind.

For a thoroughly relaxing bath, add and mix well 3 to 5 pounds of sea salt into your cold bath water. This tonic bath helps soothe aching limbs and sore muscles. Soak time is 10 to 20 minutes.

• PROVIDES RELIEF FROM SKIN DISEASES

A tub of lukewarm water fortified with a pound of baking soda is a good bath for treating skin diseases such as hives, eczema, or rashes. The mixture acts as a mild antiseptic that alleviates itching and irritation. Soak time is 10-20 minutes.

• BURNS CALORIES

A university study conducted in the UK claims that relaxing in a hot bath has health benefits equivalent to a 30-minute walk all because of the increase in body temperature.

For a calorie-burning bath, get into a tub of warm water about 104°F. Soak time is 60 minutes, so bring with you your Kindle. You may want to read about the oils that are essential in whipping up a good bath. So here they go.

THE ESSENTIAL OILS

Essential Oils are compounds pressed from barks, flowers, fruits, grasses, gums, herbs, leaves, roots, spices, and woods. They are extracted through distillation and carry the characteristic smell of the plant from where they were harvested.

Here are the more popular essential oils (with their characteristic properties) which can be used individually or in combination with other each other. Most of these oils are strong in its concentrated form and can also be used in small quantities as ingredients in homemade soaps, lotions, shampoos and other bath products.

- **Allspice**. Analgesic (relieves pain), anesthetic (causes numbness), antioxidant (protects cells against free radicals), antiseptic (fights infections), carminative (expels gas from stomach), relaxant (relieves discomfort), rubefacient (causes redness in skin due to increased blood flow to kill pain caused by musculoskeletal conditions), stimulant (stimulates the brain and central nervous system), and tonic (gives feeling of vigor or well-being).
- **Angelica**. Carminative, stimulant, tonic, antispasmodic (controls abdominal cramping), depurative (cleanses the wastes and toxins from the body), diuretic (increases urination), febrifuge (lowers fever), nervine (stimulates the nerves), and stomachic (tones the stomach and increases appetite).
- **Anise**. Antiseptic, antispasmodic, carminative, expectorant, anti-rheumatic (acts against rheumatism), sedative (reduces irritability or excitement), and vermifuge (expels intestinal parasites).
- **Basil**. Carminative, analgesic, antispasmodic, febrifuge, and antibacterial (destroys bacteria and suppresses their growth).
- Bay. Antibiotic, antispasmodic, febrifuge, sedative, stomachic, tonic, anti-neuralgic (relieves pain caused by irritation of the nerves), cholagogue (promotes bile flow into the intestines), emmenagogue (induces menstrual flow), sudorific (stimulates

sweating), insecticidal (kills insects), and astringent (evens skin tone).

- **Benzoin**. Astringent, cordial, carminative, antidepressant, disinfectant, relaxant, diuretic, anti-rheumatic, deodorant (prevents body odor caused by bacteria), vulnerary (promotes healing of wounds), and anti-inflammatory (reduces swelling).
- **Bergamot**. Antibiotic, antiseptic, antispasmodic, analgesic, antidepressant, vermifuge, and febrifuge.
- **Birch**. Antiseptic, astringent, analgesic, diuretic, febrifuge, and germicide.
- **Bitter Almond**. Anesthetic, diuretic, antispasmodic, febrifuge, sedative, bactericide, fungicide, and aperient (stimulates bowel movement). Also used in treatment of hypochondria or fear of water.
- **Black Pepper**. Digestive, carminative, aperients, antispasmodic, antirheumatic, antioxidant, and sudorific.
- **Boldo**. Anti-inflammatory, antirheumatic, cholagogue, diuretic, insecticidal, vermifuge, stimulant, and hepatic (tones or strengthens the liver).
- **Buchu**. Antiseptic, antirheumatic, carminative, digestive, diuretic, tonic, and insecticidal.
- **Cajuput**. Antiseptic, bactericide, carminative, sudorific, and decongestant (reduces swelling in the nasal passages)
- **Calamus**. Antirheumatic, antispasmodic, stimulant, memory booster, cephalic (stimulates and clears the mind), and nervine (reduces anxiety and tension).
- **Chamomile**. Antiseptic, antidepressant, carminative, cholagogue, hepatic, sudorific, stomachic, vermifuge, and vulnerary.
- **Camphor**. Antispasmodic, decongestant, sedative, antineuralgic, disinfectant, insecticidal and anesthetic.
- **Caraway**. Antiseptic, carminative, antispasmodic, stomachic, diuretic, emenagogue, expectorant, astringent, aperitif (stimulates appetite) and galactogogue (increase milk production in lactating mothers).
- **Cardamom**. Antispasmodic, antiseptic, astringent, stomachic, diuretic, aphrodisiac (arouses sexual desire). Also counters adverse effects of chemotherapy.

- **Carrot Seed**. Antiseptic, antioxidant, carminative, emmenagogue, stimulant, tonic, cytophylactic (preserves skin health).
- **Cassia**. Antidepressant, antimicrobial, antirheumatic, carminative, astringent, antiemetic (treats motion sickness), anti-diarrheal (stops or slows diarrhea).
- **Catnip**. Antispasmodic, stomachic, carminative, emmenagogue, nervine, stimulant, and astringent.
- **Cedarwood**. Antiseptic, antispasmodic, astringent, emmenagogue, expectorant, insecticidal, anti-seborrhoeic (treats seborrhea, a skin condition).
- **Cinnamon**. Antibacterial, antimicrobial, stimulant, carminative, anti-clotting (prevents blood clotting in the treatment of cardiovascular diseases).
- **Citronella**. Antidepressant, antispasmodic, deodorant, anti-inflammatory, diaphoretic, and diuretic. Also very popular as mosquito repellant.
- **Clary Sage**. Antispasmodic, aphrodisiac, carminative, deodorant, emmenagogue, nervine, stomachic, anticonvulsant (arrests epileptic seizures, euphoric (intensifies feeling of happiness and confidence).
- **Clove**. Antimicrobial, antifungal, aphrodisiac, and antiseptic.
- **Coriander**. Antispasmodic, analgesic, aphrodisiac, carminative, stomachic, lipolytic (melts unwanted fatty deposits).
- **Cumin**. Bactericidal, digestive, carminative, antiseptic, antispasmodic, diuretic, emmenagogue, nervice and tonic.
- **Cypress**. Astringent, antispasmodic, antiseptic, hepatic, deodorant, sudorific, sedative, respiratory tonic, hemostatic (arrests hemorrhaging), styptic (stops bleeding when applied on wounds).
- **Davana**. Antidepressant, antiviral, emmenagogue, expectorant, antiseptic, relaxant, and vulnerary.
- **Dill**. Antispasmodic, digestive, carminative, galactagogue, sedative, sudorific, and stomachic.
- **Elemi**. Antiseptic, expectorant, analgesic, stimulant and tonic.
- **Eucalyptus**. Anti-inflammatory, decongestant, deodorant, antiseptic, antispasmodic, stimulant.

- **Fennel**. Antiseptic, aperitif, carminative, diuretic, emmenagogue, galactogogue, stomachic, tonic, vermifuge, and depurative.
- **Frankincense**. Antiseptic, astringent, carminative, cicatrisant, diuretic, expectorant, sedative, tonic, vulnerary, uterine (promotes healthy uterus)
- **Galbanum**. Antirheumatic, antispasmodic, decongestant, antioxidant, insecticidal, vulnerary, anti-parasitic, emollient (promotes supple skin).
- **Geranium**. Astringent, cicatrisant, diuretic, styptic, diuretic, tonic, and vulnerary.
- **Ginger**. Antiseptic, antispasmodic, carminative, expectorant, cephalic, rubefacient, stomachic, and anti-emetic (arrests vomiting and nausea).
- **Grapefruit**. Diuretic, stimulant, disinfectant, antidepressant, aperitif and tonic.
- **Helichrysum**. Antispasmodic, nervine, anti-inflammatory, expectorant, hepatic, mucolytic (thins mucus making it easier to cough up), and ant-tusive (suppresses cough).
- **Hyssop**. Stimulant, antiseptic, carminative, diuretic, astringent, nervine, sudorific, vermifuge, vulnerary, and tonic.
- **Jasmine**. Antiseptic, antispasmodic, expectorant, emmenagogue, galactagogue, uterine, and sedative.
- **Juniper**. Antiseptic, antirheumatic, antispasmodic, stomachic, carminative, rubefacient, astringent, sudorific, and tonic.
- **Lavandin**. Antidepressant, analgesic, antiseptic, expectorant, vulnerary, nervine, and cicatrisant.
- **Lavender**. Analgesic, disinfectant, antiseptic, anti-inflammatory, and sleep-inducing.
- **Lemon**. Antiseptic, astringent, disinfectant, febrifuge, tonic, and restorative (arrests depression and mental, emotional, and muscular tension).
- **Lemongrass**. Analgesic, antimicrobial, antiseptic, carminative, antiseptic, deodorant, diuretic, galactogogue, nervine, sedative, and tonic.
- **Lime**. Antiseptic, astringent, antiviral, febrifuge, restorative, and tonic.
- **Mandarin**. Antiseptic, cytophylactic, depurative, hepatic, relaxant, stomachic and tonic.

- **Manuka**. Anti-dandruff, antibacterial, anti-inflammatory, deodorant, anti-allergic, relaxant, antidote to insect bites.
- **Marjoram**. Analgesic, antiseptic, bactericidal, cephalic, carminative, cordial, digestive, expectorant, laxative, nervice, stomachic, vulnerary, and a vasodilator (relaxes the smooth nerve muscles causing the vessels to dilate and consequently lower blood pressure).
- **Melissa**. Antidepressant, nervie, cordial, sedative, stomachic, carminative, febrifuge, sudorific, tonic, hypotensive (lowers blood pressure), and diaphoretic (induces heavy sweating).
- **Mugwort**. Cordial, diuretic, nervine, stimulant, vermifuge, and uterine.
- **Mullein**. Analgesic, antiseptic, diuretic, febrifuge, expectorant, and relaxant.
- **Mustard**. Stimulant, aperitif, antifungal, cordial, insect repellant, and tonic.
- **Myrrh**. Antimicrobial, expectorant, astringent, carminative, stomachic, diaphoretic, tonic, and anti-catarrhal (removes excess mucus due to infection of the ears, nose, and throat).
- **Myrtle**. Antiseptic, deodorant, sedative, astringent, and expectorant.
- **Neroli**. Antidepressant, antiseptic, cordial, carminative, antispasmodic, emollient, deodorant, and tonic.
- **Niaouli**. Analgesic, antiseptic, decongestant, febrifuge, insecticidal, vermifuge, vulnerary, and balsamic (softens mucus).
- **Nutmeg**. Analgesic, antioxidant, antiseptic, anti-parasitic, aphrodisiac, laxative, stimulant, antiemetic, and tonic.
- **Oakmoss**. Antiseptic, expectorant, restorative, and demulcent (forms a oral protective film for relief from irritation of the mucous membranes lining the inside of the mouth).
- **Orange**. Anti-inflammatory, antispasmodic, carminative, sedative, diuretic, cholagogue, and tonic.
- **Oregano**. Antiviral, anti-fungal, digestive, antioxidant, and anti-allergenic.
- **Palma Rosa**. Antiseptic, cytophylactic, febrifuge, digestive, and antiviral.
- **Parsley**. Antimicrobial, antiseptic, carminative, astringent, diuretic, laxative, hypotensive, stomachic and uterine.

- **Patchouli**. Antidepressant, antiseptic, astringent, cytophylactic, diuretic, deodorant, febrifuge, sedative, and anti-inflammatory.
- **Pennyroyal**. Antimicrobial, antirheumatic, antiseptic, cordial, astringent, depurative, emmenagogue, decongestant, and stomachic.
- **Peppermint**. Analgesic, antiseptic, antispasmodic, anti-inflammatory, expectorant, hepatic, stomachic, sudorific, vermifuge, and vasoconstrictor (causes the smooth nerve muscles to contract in order to stop hemorrhaging).
- **Petitgrain**. Antiseptic, antispasmodic, deodorant, sedative, and nervine.
- **Pimento**. Anesthetic, antioxidant, carminative, stimulant, and tonic.
- **Pine**. Antibacterial, diuretic, antiseptic, and analgesic.
- **Ravensara**. Analgesic, antibacterial, antifungal, antispasmodic, expectorant, relaxant, and tonic.
- **Rose**. Antidepressant, antiseptic, aphrodisiac, cholagogue, depurative, cicatrisant, hepatic, nervine, laxative, stomachic, uterine.
- **Rosemary**. Disinfectant, anti-inflammatory, antibacterial, analgesic, and carminative. Also promotes hair growth.
- **Rosewood**. Analgesic, antiseptic, cephalic, insecticidal, deodorant, and stimulant.
- **Rue**. Antirheumatic, antifungal, and insecticidal.
- **Sage**. Antifungal, antiseptic, anti-inflammatory, antispasmodic, cicatrisant, digestive, febrifuge, laxative, stimulant, and choleretic (increaseas volume of bile secretion necessary for digestion of fats).
- **Sandalwood**. Antiseptic, antiphlogistic, astringent, carminative, cicatrisant, diuretic, emollient, hypotensive, tonic, and a memory booster.
- **Spearmint**. Antiseptic, carminative, antispasmodic, emmenagogue, restorative, insecticidal, and stimulating.
- **Spikenard**. Anti-inflammatory, antibacterial, deodorant, laxative, sedative, and uterine.
- **Tagetes**. Antimicrobial, antiseptic, disinfectant, sedative, insecticidal, antispasmodic, and anti-parasitic.

- **Tangerine**. Antispasmodic, antiseptic, depurative, cytophylactic, sedative, stomachic and tonic.
- **Tansy**. Antifungal, anti-inflammatory, cytophylactic, stomachic, and tonic.
- **Tarragon**. Antirheumatic, digestive, emmenagogue, stimulant, deodorant, and vermifuge.
- **Tea Tree**. Antimicrobial, insecticidal, balsamic, expectorant, sudorific, and stimulant.
- **Thuja**. Antirheumatic, diuretic, expectorant, rubefacient, astringent, vermifuge, stimulant, and tonic.
- **Thyme**. Antispasmodic, antiseptic, carminative, diuretic, expectorant, insecticidal, stimulant, vermifugal, and tonic.
- **Tuberose**. Deodorant, sedative, and aphrodisiac.
- **Vanilla**. Antioxidant, anti-carcinogenic, antidepressant, and sedative.
- **Vetiver**. Anti-inflammatory, cicatrisant, sedative, nervine, and tonic.
- **Wintergreen**. Analgesic, antrheumatic, antispasmodic, astringent, diuretic, carminative, stimulant, and anodyne (allays pain).
- **Wormwood**. Deodorant, emmenagogue, insecticidal, vermifuge, and tonic.
- **Yarrow**. Anti-inflammatory, antiseptic, astringent, antispasmodic, carminative, diaphoretic, hypotensive, stomachic, and tonic.
- **Ylang-ylang**. Antidepressant, antiseptic, and anti-seborrhoeic.

These essential oils are usually diluted in carrier oils when used in aromatherapy

AROMATHERAPY

Aromatherapy is the use of diluted essential oils extracted from plants for physical and physiological well-being. It may be offered as a complementary therapy alongside standard medical treatment; or altogether a form of alternative medicine.

YOU GAIN THE BENEFITS OF AROMATHERAPY IN 3 WAYS:

- **Through the sense of smell.** Some of your best memories are tied to particular smells. Inhalation of aromatic oil molecules stimulates olfactory nerves in the nose that send signals to the brain. Depending on the emotions triggered, the process inevitably affects your mood.
- **Absorption via the respiratory system.** You reap the antiviral and antibacterial properties of aromatic oils through inhalation. The aromatic oil molecules travel to the sinuses, throat and air passageways which help alleviate infections and allergies.
- **Absorption through the skin.** The moment aromatic oil molecules permeate the skin, you begin to reap the benefits of its antiviral, antibacterial, antioxidant, anti-aging, and antidepressant properties.

Aromatic oils used in aromatherapy are usually 2% essential oils diluted in 98% carrier oils like grape seed, almond oil, and skin care oil. In baths, you would usually mix the essential oil of your choice plus the carrier oil with your bath water.

AROMATHERAPY FOR YOUR BATHS

An aromatherapy bath is a good way for essential oils to do wonders to your body leaving you relaxed and rejuvenated. It also keeps your skin supple.

To get the most out of your aromatherapy oils and to experience the benefits of a good bath, here's a guide:

• *Know your oils and quantities.*
  - 1 teaspoon of carrier oil such as avocado oil, almond oil, grape seed oil, or apricot oil.
  - 5 drops of essential oil that you choose based on the purpose of your bath. You may refer to the enumeration of essential oils above; or you may check the recommendations below:
    - For a sensuous bath, try sandalwood, ylang-ylang, neroli, jasmine, or rose.
    - For skin-soothing baths, you may try chamomile, lavender, patchouli, or sandalwood.
    - If you have trouble sleeping, try marjoram or sandalwood.
    - There are essential oils that are not bath-friendly, so it is always best to read essential oil labels. The following oils are to be avoided: pimenta, nutmeg, clove, black pepper, oregano, thyme, cinnamon, and basil.
    - Check labels as well if your essential oil won't have adverse effects on pregnant or breastfeeding moms, children, and the elderly.
  - Mix the carrier oil and essential oils together before incorporating them into your water. Never mix pure, undiluted essential oils directly into your bath water as they may irritate your skin.

• *Check the temperature of your water.*
    - 70-80°F for a stimulating cold bath. Soaking time is 2-5 minutes.
    - 80-93°F for a relaxing warm bath. Soaking time is at least 20 minutes.
    - 100-104°F for healing and detoxing hot bath. Soak until you

feel relief from say your colds or flue, or if you feel that you're done with excessive sweating.

• *Set the right ambience.*
- Light aromatherapy candles.
- Dim the lights.
- Play soft music.
- Bring a favorite bath pillow.
- Sprinkle rose petals in your tub.

ALL ABOUT BATH SOAPS AND SOAP MAKING

Soap making can be likened to painting where your palette of colors is the array of ingredients you can use, each with different characteristic properties. Taking into consideration their individual qualities will allow you to create your masterpiece soap recipe.

Soap comes as a result of mixing **lye (sodium hydroxide or caustic soda)** dissolved in water and a specific amount of oils. Lye is sold in different forms: flakes, beads, pellets, powder or liquid. When lye water and heated oils are mixed, a chemical reaction occurs in a process called **saponification.** Careful measurements of ingredients results to a well-balanced bar of soap. Too much lye and the soap's PH will be too high and will cause itchiness on the skin. On the other hand, too little lye will result in a soft and greasy soap that may not set at all. For this reason, it's important to use a lye calculator. You can easily download a portable **Lye Calculator** from your App Store. A lye calculator comes handy in determining how much lye you need in your recipe and how big your finished batch will be.

Every oil has what is called **saponification value or SAP**. This number indicates the amount of lye water needed to turn 1 gram of oil into soap. Therefore, changing the amount of one oil in your recipe would require you to go through the lye calculator all over again to re-compute measurements for the entire ingredients list.

Use only fresh oils so you don't get the **Dreaded Orange Spots** or **DOS** on you soap. They are unsightly and leave you with a rancid product.

Superfat (or **Lye Discount**) is the amount of oil that you put in your recipe that is beyond the amount of lye that's available to turn your mixture into soap.   So if for example you indicated a superfat of 5% (the percentage generally recommended), it only means that 5% of the oils in your recipe will not saponifiy, leaving you with a bar of soap with extra oil to nourish your skin some more. A superfat of 10% is the highest most soap makers would suggest. Any percentage higher would result to a soggy product. Also, too much oil free-floating on your bar would inhibit lathering.

Trace is that stage in the soap making process at which lye water and the oils start to combine together to make the soap. When the mixture turns to the consistency of pudding, this means the mixture has gone into thin to medium trace. This is the time to add your fragrances, additives, and colorants.

After the fragrances are mixed in, you may now pour your soap in a mold. Your soap will harden overnight.   If your soap cools too quickly, you'd find that **soda ash** has formed on the surface the following day. It is a whitish powder that should not be cause for concern.   It is not harmful on the skin and your soap can still be used. All you need to do wash it off under cold water or scrape it off with a knife.

Your soap is not ready for use until after it undergoes **curing** for 4 to 6 weeks.

OILS FOR SOAP MAKING

- **FOR HARD AND LONG LASTING SOAPS**
  - **Lard**. Lard turns out super-hard immaculately white soap bars with a stable, creamy lather. It would create less foamy suds but the moisturizing effect is remarkable. Combining lard with the reliable olive and coconut oils makes a balanced bar of soap that is easy on the budget. Be wary though that the lard you buy is fresh and of good quality, lest you get that greasy scent on your soap. Use only a percentage of lard not more than 40% in your soap recipe.
  - **Beef Tallow**. Beef Tallow, which appears as sodium tallowate in product labels, is an animal oil perfect in combination with coconut and olive oils. The result is a soap concoction you'd love for its heavy and creamy lather which you won't find in non-tallow soaps. The percentage of tallow in your soap recipe should not be more than 40%.

- **FOR LATHERY SOAPS**
  - **Babassu Oil**. Babassu oil is extracted from the seeds of the babassu palm. It is rich in myristic and lauric acid that's perfect if you want your soap to produce abundant fluffy lather.
  - **Castor Oil**. Castor oil is viscous, clear oil that is perfect for increasing the lathering properties of your soap. About 8% of castor oil in your soap recipe promises rich, creamy soap suds that would leave your skin highly moisturized. Use only about 5% - 8% of castor oil in your soap recipe.
  - **Coconut Oil.** Coconut oil is undoubtedly one of the most popular oils used in soap recipes to achieve a marvelous rich lather. Using 30% of coconut oil in your recipe makes your soap a superb cleansing agent for stripping your body of excess skin oil.

- **FOR MOISTURIZING SOAPS**
  - **Avocado Oil.** Avocado oil is green oil that doesn't readily react with lye to form soap. For this reason, it is a good option to superfat with. Its highly moisturizing properties make it a good ingredient for soaps intended for use by people with sensitive skin. Use from 5%-30% of avocado oil in your soap recipes.
  - **Canola Oil.** Canola is a cheaper substitute for olive oil. It has properties that slow down tracing, so it's good to add canola into your recipe if you plan to do complicated designs with your soap. Use 10%-15% of canola in your soap recipe for a nice, creamy lather.
  - **Grapeseed Oil.** Grapeseed oil is a light moisturizing oil that is a good ingredient to your soap because it gets absorbed into the skin really well, so you feel moisturized without the greasy after-feel. Use only at most 5% in your recipe.
  - **Hazelnut Oil.** Hazelnut oil is a first-rate moisturizer but it has a very short shelf life. An old stock added to your mixture may cause DOS. Use only 5%-10% of hazelnut oil in your soap recipe.
  - **Extra Virgin Olive Oil**. Extra virgin olive oil is the extract collected from the first pressing of the olives. The well-known Castille soap is made from 100% olive oil. Soaps made with olive oil are hard and white and are excellent moisturizers. Olive oil is best combined with other oils for richer lather.
  - **Rice Bran Oil.** Rice bran oil, expressed from the husks of milled rice, is the budget-friendly substitute for olive oil. When included in your soap recipe, it gives the same moisturizing properties that olive oil does. Rice bran oil also has the same vitamins and antioxidants present in olive oil.
  - **Sesame Seed Oil.** Almost everyone is familiar with the characteristic scent of sesame oil. It is rich in vitamins and antioxidants making it a good additive to your soap recipe for a highly moisturizing and conditioning concoction.
  - **Liquid Soybean Oil.** Soybean oil works well in combination with primary oils like coconut, palm, and olive. You may use 5%-15% of this oil for your soap recipe. It may result to a soap that gives low, creamy lather, but you'll love the mildness and

the moisturizing wonder. Soybean oil is a readily available and cheaper alternative for making big batches of soap making it popular among budget-conscious soap makers.

- **Soybean Oil Shortening**. Soybean oil, when hydrogenated, is commonly called vegetable shortening. Shortening is usually a mix of soybean and cottonseed oil and is a common soap recipe ingredient.   It combines well with coconut and olive oils resulting to soaps that are stable, foamy, and highly moisturizing.
- **Sunflower Oil.** Sunflower oil, when combined with olive and palm oils results into soaps that give the richest creamy lather well-loved for its moisturizing effect. Limit to about 25% of sunflower oil in your soap recipes for good results.

• FOR A LUXURIOUS SUPER MOISTURIZING SOAP

- **Sweet Almond Oil.** Sweet almond oil is moisturizing oil desired for its very light property. Including about 5%-10% of sweet almond oil in your soap recipe gives you a bar that produces low but stable lather.
- **Apricot Kernel Oil.** Apricot kernel oil, similar to the makeup of almond oil, is a light oil that gets absorbed really well into the skin; and its excellent conditioning property leaves you supple all over. Use only 5%-10% of apricot kernel oil in your soap recipes.
- **Hemp Seed Oil.**   Hemp seed oil is greenish oil with a nutty smell.   Including hemp seed oil in your recipe provides you a soap that gives a light, silky lather. Use 10%-15% of this oil in your soap recipes for a luxurious bath.
- **Jojoba Oil.**   Jojoba is a liquid wax comparable to sebum in chemical composition. When added to your soap recipe, it contributes to a rich stable lather with moisturizing qualities that's readily absorbed into the skin. It causes the soap mixture to trace rapidly, so it isn't a good choice for soaps intended for complex designs, swirls, and colorings. Use only 5%-10% of jojoba oil in your soap recipes.

- **FOR HEALING SOAPS**
  - **Kukui Nut Oil.**   Oil extracted from the kukui nut is a good ingredient for making soaps with high lathering property. A soap made with kukui oil moisturizes skin well and is supposed to give relief from acne, psoriasis and eczema.   In your soap recipe, use about 5%-10% of kukui oil.
  - **Neem Oil.**   Neem oil, known for its anti-fungal and antiseptic properties, is extracted from the bark of the neem tree. Neem oil scent may be strong but it's nutty smell blends perfectly with earthy fragrances. Using about 25% of neem oil in your soap recipe makes it a good agent for treating athlete's foot and other skin ailments.
  - **Pumpkin Seed Oil.**   Pumpkin seed oil is a premium oil that's jam-packed with Vitamins A, C, E, and Omega-3 fatty acid making it an effective antioxidant.   Pumpkin seed oil is, therefore, a must-have ingredient for making soaps intended for optimum skin care.
  - **Wheatgerm Oil.**   Wheatgerm oil's amber to reddish brown color is an indication that it is rich in Vitamin E. This sticky oil helps stimulate the antioxidant properties of the other oils included in the recipe. Just 15% of wheatgerm oil added into the soap concoction is enough for a superb healing bath experience.

HOMEMADE SOAP RECIPES

With soap making, you'd be handling corrosive materials so you should gear up for safety. Always wear goggles, gloves and long sleeves. Also, make sure that your kids and pets are restricted from entering your soap making space. Your work area should be well-ventilated and are rid of distractions and tripping hazards.

Now, if you wouldn't want to work with lye, there are readily available melt-and-pour soap bases like goat milk soap that you can shove into your microwave and is ready for use with the other ingredients in your recipe in a few seconds. It's like making cake using cake mix so you can't really call it your own personalized concoction.

1. THE STARTER 3-OIL SOAP

Ingredients:

Will make a 2-pound batch

- 6 ounces coconut oil
- 9.4 ounces Crisco
- 6 ounces olive oil
- 7 ounces water
- 0.9 ounces essential oil
- 3 ounces lye

Preparation:

1. Prepare the lye solution. Let it cool.

2. Melt the solid oils.

3. Add the liquid oils into the melted solid oils effectively lowering its temperature.

4. As soon as the lye solution and the oils cool down to 120°F, gently pour the solution into the oils. Stir using a stick blender.

5. Continue blending and stirring until the soap gets to thin trace.

6. Add in fragrance or colorants. Mix with a whisk. At this point you may not use your stick blender anymore in agitating the mixture.

7. Transfer soap into a mold. Let sit for 24-36 hours or until the soap is hard enough for cutting.

8. Remove the soap from the mold and cut into bars.

9. Arrange bars in a tray making sure that they touch each other.

10.   Cure for 2 to 4 weeks.

2. CHARCOAL FACIAL SOAP

Ingredients:
- 14.4 ounces olive oil (40%)
- 9 ounces coconut oil (25%)
- 9 ounces palm oil (25%)
- 1.8 ounces castor oil (5%)
- 1.8 ounces tamanu oil (5%)
- 10.1 ounces distilled water
- 5.1 ounces lye
- 1.7 ounces tea tree essential oil
- 2 tablespoons activated charcoal
- 12-bar rectangle silicone mold

Procedure:
1. Add lye to the water. Stir well until all the lye has completely dissolved and the liquid is already clear.

2. Melt the solid oils: olive, coconut, palm, and castor. Only after melting the oils could you do portioning. Then mix the oils together.

3. Once the temperatures of the lye water and the oils have gone down to 120°F (or are within 10° of each other), mix the oils with the lye water and stir using a stick blender until the soap gets to thin trace.

4. Fold in the activated charcoal into the soap. Only then can you slowly incorporate the charcoal into the batter using the stick blender at pulse setting.

5. Add the tea tree oil and continue stick blending until the oil is completely blended in. Continue stick blending for a few more seconds until medium trace.

6. Pour the soap into a rectangular mold. Gently tap the mold on your countertop to remove bubbles.

7. Spritz the surface of the soap with 99% isopropyl alcohol to prevent formation of soda ash.

8. Place the mold on a heating pad set to medium. Insulate the soap (cover the mold with a lid or piece of cardboard) and let it sit for 30 minutes. Afterwards, turn the heating pad off and, without removing the insulation, leave the mold on it for the 24 hours.

9. Let the soap stay in the mold from 3 days to a week. You may unmold when the soap is already firm.

10. Cure for 4 to 6 weeks.

3. ALOE VERA SOAP

Ingredients:
- 3 ounces lye
- 7.5 ounces distilled water
- 1.8 ounces aloe vera juice
- 0.4 ounces beeswax
- 1.5 pounds extra virgin olive oil
- 0.18 ounces mint essential oil

Procedure:

1. Prepare your lye water by mixing lye with water in a stainless steel container. Let cool to about 120°F.

2. In a separate pan, melt the olive oil while gradually mixing in the beeswax. Remove from heat and allow to cool down to the same temperature as the lye solution.

3. Mix the lye water with the oil mixture and stick blend until medium trace.

4. Pour in the mint essential oil and aloe vera juice. Whisk the mixture for a minute more.

5. Pour the soap in molds. Gently tap the mold on your countertop to remove bubbles.

6. Insulate your soap for 2 days. Then air for a day. Remove the soap from its mold and cut into bars. Arrange the bars on a tray lined with wax paper.

7. Cure for 4 weeks. Turn the bars occasionally to dry uniformly.

4. LAVENDER-OATMEAL SOAP

Ingredients:
- 10 ounces melt-and-pour goat milk soap (as base)
- ¼ teaspoon lavender essential oil
- ¼ cup oatmeal
- 1 tablespoon lavender flowers, dried

Procedure:

1. Chop the goat milk soap into chunks. Place the chunks in a microwaveable container. Add in the oats and lavender flowers.

2. Microwave for over a minute to melt. Mix in the lavender essential oil and stir well. Pour into molds.

3. Allow the mixture to cool until hard before unmolding your lavender-oatmeal soap.

4. You may refrigerate to chill them, but do not freeze.

5. GRAPEFRUIT IN PINK HIMALAYAN SALT SOAP

Ingredients:
- 1 pound melt-and-pour goat milk soap (as base)
- 10-15 drops grapefruit essential oil
- ¼ cup pink himalayan salt

Preparation:

1. In a double boiler, melt the goat milk soap.

2. Remove melted soap from heat. Mix in grapefruit essential oil.

3. Add in pink himalayan salt and quickly pour into molds.

4. Let the soap harden for at least 2 hours, then you may unmold.

6. COFFEE SOAP

Ingredients:
- 1-½ pounds melt-and-pour goat milk soap (as base)
- 1 teaspoon almond oil
- 1 tablespoon freshly-ground coffee

Procedure:

1. Cut the soap base into chunks. Using a double boiler, melt the chunks over medium-low flame.

2. Remove from heat. Quickly add the ground coffee and almond oil. Mix well.

3. Pour into the molds short of the top. Spritz with isopropyl alcohol to prevent bubbles from forming.

4. As soon the soap hardens, pop them out from the molds. They are ready for use. No curing is needed.

5. Store in airtight containers.

7. MOCHA SOAP

Ingredients:
- 1 teaspoon cocoa powder
- 6 ounces double-strength coffee
- 2.4 ounces lye
- 2 ounces grapeseed oil
- 1 ounces palm kennel oil
- 4 ounces palm oil
- 4 ounces coconut oil

Procedure:

1. Mix lye and double-strength coffee.

2. Melt the oils in a double boiler.

3. Pour the lye mixture into the melted oils and mix with a stick blender.

4. At light trace, add the cocoa powder and continue stick blending until fully incorporated and no clumps are visible.

5. Pour the mixture into a mold. Insulate the mold with a towel and let sit for 48 hours.

6. Unmold the soap, cut into bars and arrange in a baking sheet lined with wax paper.

7. Cure for 4 weeks minimum.

8. SILK SOAP

Ingredients:
- 4.37 ounces lye
- 12.06 ounces distilled water
- 3.18 ounces castor oil
- 12.7 ounces olive oil
- 7.9 ounces shea butter
- 7.9 ounces coconut oil
- 0.6 ounces silk peptide

Additives:
- 0.6 ounces fragrance of your choice
- ½ teaspoon soap color, dark pink
- ½ teaspoon soap color, yellow
- ½ teaspoon soap color, orange
- ½ teaspoon white mica
- 2 teaspoons kaolin clay
- 4 tablespoons olive oil, divided

Procedure:

1. Prepare the colorants by portioning the olive oil into glasses. To each glass, add the kaolin clay and each of the 3 colorants.

2. Using a spoon, mix thoroughly each olive oil-colorant and oil-clay mixture into a paste. Set aside.

3. Prepare your lye water. Add in the silk peptide. The lye water may turn a golden yellow. Set aside.

4. Place all the oils into a bowl. Pour in the silk-lye water mixture. Mix vigorously until all the oils have melted.

5. Add in the soft oils and mix using a stick blender until light trace. Incorporate the fragrance at this time.

6. Apportion your soap into the four glasses containing the olive oil-colorants and oil-kaolin clay mixtures. Mix thoroughly.

7. Pour each colored soap into individual squeeze bottles. Squeeze the colored soap into a mold. Remember to alternate between colors.

8. Insulate for 48 hours, then cut into bars.

9. Arrange in a baking sheet lined with wax paper.

10. Cure for 4 weeks.

9. SPOON SWIRL

Ingredients:
- 4.6 ounces lye
- 12.06 ounces distilled water
- 7.94 ounces palm oil
- 1.59 ounces castor oil
- 12.7 ounces olive oil
- 9.52 ounces coconut oil

Additives:
- 1-¼ teaspoon white mica, divided
- ¼ teaspoon yellow oxide
- ¼ teaspoon black oxide
- ¼ teaspoon cocoa powder

Procedure:

1. Add lye into distilled water.

2. Melt the solid oils in a double boiler.

3. Combine the lye water and melted oils. Bring to thin trace.

4. Apportion the soap into four glasses, one glass for each of the colorants:

   - Glass A – ½ teaspoon white mica
   - Glass B – ¼ teaspoon yellow oxide + ¼ teaspoon white mica
   - Glass C – ¼ teaspoon black oxide + ¼ teaspoon white mica
   - Glass D – ¼ teaspoon cocoa powder + ¼ teaspoon white mica

5. Mix a quarter portion of the soap in each color and blend together well.

6. Drizzle the colored soaps alternatingly into the mold until all the soaps are all used up. If the soaps thicken a little while you are doing all the drizzling, just give the mixture a little stir.

7. Once the mold is full, insulate with a towel and leave it to set overnight.   Then cut into bars.

8. Cure for 4 weeks.

10. VEGAN SOAP

Ingredients:
- 4.5 ounces lye
- 10 ounces distilled water
- 4 ounces shea butter
- 4 ounces almond oil
- 6 ounces avocado oil
- 8 ounces palm oil
- 10 ounces coconut oil

Procedure:

1. Prepare your lye water by combining lye with distilled water. Set aside and let cool down.

2. In a double boiler, melt the oils. Then add in the lye water. Give the solution a brief stir then continue stirring using with a stick blender.

3. As soon the soap gets to thin trace, cover the double boiler and let the soap set for an hour.

4. Transfer the soap into your mold and insulate overnight.

5. Unmold and cut into bars.

6. Arrange on a baking sheet line with wax paper.

7. Cure for 2-4 weeks.

SHAMPOOS

Make everyday a great hair day with any of the following shampoo recipes. There's always a right recipe for your every hair need.

1. SHAMPOO FOR NORMAL HAIR

Ingredients:
- ¼ cup liquid Castile Soap (any variant)
- ¼ cup distilled water
- ½ teaspoon grapeseed or jojoba oil
- Use a foaming bottle or flip-cap bottle for storage and dispensing

Procedure:

Mix all ingredients together and store in a dispenser. Shake well before use. Although not as thick as shampoos available commercially, this basic shampoo mixture produces great lather.

2. SHAMPOO FOR STIMULATING SCALP

Ingredients:
- ¼ cup Castile Soap (unscented)
- ¼ cup distilled water
- 1/8 teaspoon peppermint oil
- ½ teaspoon jojoba oil
- 1/8 teaspoon tea tree essential oil
- Use a foaming bottle or flip-cap bottle for storage and dispensing

Procedure:

Mix all ingredients together and store in a dispenser. Use like you would any shampoo. Rinse well.

3. MOISTURIZING SHAMPOO FOR DRY HAIR

Ingredients:
- ¼ cup liquid Castile Soap (any variant)
- ¼ cup distilled water
- 1 teaspoon glycerin
- ¼ cup aloe vera gel
- ¼ teaspoon avocado or jojoba oil
- Use a foaming bottle or flip-cap bottle as dispenser

Procedure:

Mix well all the ingredients and store in a dispenser. Shake well before every use. Apply generously to hair and let sit for a few minutes. Rinse well under cool water.

4. SOOTHING SHAMPOO TO CALM YOUR NERVES

Ingredients:
- 1 cup Castille Soap (Lavender)
- 1 cup distilled water
- 1-1/2 tablespoons glycerin
- 6 chamomile tea bags
- Use a flip-cap bottle for storage and dispensing

Procedure:

Let the chamomile teabags steep in a cup of hot water for 20 minutes. Then discard the tea bags. Stir in Castille soap and glycerin and mix well. Transfer in a dispenser and store in a cool, dark place.

5. ANTI-DANDRUFF SHAMPOO

Ingredients:
- ¼ cup Castile Soap
- ¼ cup distilled water
- 1 tablespoon apple cider vinegar
- ¼ teaspoon jojoba or grapeseed oil
- 6 cloves, finely ground
- 3 tablespoons apple juice
- Use a foaming bottle or flip-cap bottle for storage and dispensing

Procedure:

In a blender, mix all the ingredients on low setting for 30 seconds and store in the refrigerator.   Wet hair with warm water and shampoo the mixture into hair and massage thoroughly. Discard leftovers after 3 days.

6.   SHINE SHAMPOO

Ingredients:
- ¼ cup liquid Castile soap (Lemon)
- ¼ cup distilled water
- 2 tablespoons almond oil
- 2 tablespoons dried rosemary
- ¼ teaspoon lemon essential oil
- Use a foaming bottle or flip-cap bottle for storage and dispensing

Procedure:

Add rosemary in boiled distilled water and let steep until aroma is released. Run through a strainer and let coll. Mix in all the other ingredients and add a little water before stirring. Transfer into a dispenser. Use like you would any shampoo. Rinse well under cool water.

7. TEA TREE AND ROSEMARY SHAMPOO FOR ALL HAIR TYPES

Ingredients:
- ¼ cup Castile Soap (any variant)
- ¼ cup distilled water
- 2 teaspoon tea tree oil
- 3 tablespoons rosemary
- 2 tablespoon lemongrass
- 1 teaspoon vanilla essential oil
- ½ teaspoon grapeseed oil or jojoba oil
- Use a foaming bottle or flip-cap bottle for storage and dispensing

Procedure:

Put lemongrass and rosemary in a tea strainer and let steep in boiled distilled water for 30 minutes until aroma is released. Discard the leaves and let cool. Mix in all the other ingredients, add a little water and mix some more. Mix in vanilla and tea tree oil. Let the shampoo cool and transfer into the dispenser. Use like you would any shampoo. Rinse well under cold water.

8. COCONUT SHAMPOO FOR SHINY HAIR

Ingredients:
- ¼ cup liquid Castile Soap (unscented)
- ¼ cup distilled water
- 10 drops coconut fragrance oil
- 10 drops vanilla essential oil
- 2 teaspoons jojoba oil
- Use a foaming bottle or flip-cap bottle for storage and dispensing

Procedure:

Mix all ingredients together. Transfer in a dispenser. Use like you would any shampoo. Rinse well with cool water.

9. DRY SHAMPOO

Ingredients:
- 1 teaspoon lavender (or any fragrant herb)
- ¼ cup cornstarch (or for dark hair, cocoa powder)
- Recycled container with a sprinkle top

Procedure:

Mix the ingredients and transfer into the container. Sprinkle generously to cover hair. Spread evenly using a comb. Store leftovers in a cool, dry place.

10. ROSEMARY PALE ALE SHAMPOO BAR

Ingredients:
- 1 pound Castile Soap (any variant), shredded
- ½ cup + 2 tablespoons pale ale
- 1 tablespoon jojoba oil
- 2 teaspoons rosemary essential oil
- 1 tablespoon avocado oil
- 2 tablespoons kaolin or rhassoul clay
- Wooden or silicon molds

Procedure:

Grate the Castille soap. Combine grated soap with the half cup of pale ale in a crack pot on low setting. Melt the mixture. In a bowl, mix together the clay and 2 tablespoons pale ale. Stir the jojoba oil, rosemary essential oil, and avocado oil into the clay mixture. Transfer the final mixture into a mold lined with parchment paper. Leave it to harden for 3 days. Remove from the mold and cut into bars. To use, wet hair. Form a rich lather out of the shampoo bar and apply to hair and massage into scalp. Rinse well.

11. RYE FLOUR SHAMPOO

Ingredients:
- 3 tablespoons organic rye flour
- ½ cup distilled water

Procedure:

Mix water and rye to form a runny paste.   Rub the mixture evenly onto scalp and let sit for a couple of minutes.   Rinse off with warm water.

12. KIDDIE SHAMPOO

Ingredients:
- ¼ cup Castile Soap (any variant)
- ½ cup distilled water
- 10 drops melaleuca essential oil
- 8 drops lemon essential oil
- Reuse an empty shampoo bottle for storage and dispensing

Procedure:

Mix all ingredients in a bowl and transfer into the reusable bottle for storage. To use, shake well and pour a small portion into palm. Massage into scalp and work down through the hair. Rinse well.

13. HONEY-COCONUT SHAMPOO

Ingredients:
- ½ cup Castille soap (any variant)
- 1 tablespoon Vitamin E oil
- ¼ cup coconut milk
- ¼ cup honey
- 2 tablespoons jojoba oil
- 30-40 drops essential oil
- Recycled shampoo bottle for storage and dispensing

Procedure:

Mix all the ingredients in an empty shampoo bottle. Shake well before every use.

14. BAKING SODA SHAMPOO

Ingredients:
- 1 cup distilled water
- 1 tablespoon baking soda
- Recycled shampoo bottle

Procedure:

Fill the shampoo bottle with water. Add in the baking soda. Shake well before use. To use, squirt a little amount onto wet hair. Massage thoroughly and let sit for a few minutes. Make sure to rinse well.

15. EGG SHAMPOO FOR OILY HAIR

Ingredients:
- 2 teaspoons lemon juice (or vinegar)
- 2 egg yolks
- Essential oil to neutralize the eggy smell

Procedure:

Blend together the yolks, lemon juice, and essential oil. Rub the mixture onto wet hair. Rinse well under cool water.

16. ALOE VERA SHAMPOO FOR STRONG LONG HAIR

Ingredients:
- ¼ cup Castile Soap
- ¼ cup Aloe Vera juice
- 2 capsules Vitamin E oil
- 5 drops Lavender essential oil
- Recycled shampoo bottle

Procedure:

In a mixing bowl, blend together the Castile soap, Aloe vera juice, and lavender oil.   Puncture the Vitamin E capsules and squeeze out the contents into the mix. Mix some more. Transfer the mixture into the shampoo bottle and store in the refrigerator. To use, pour a small amount onto wet hair and massage to form a rich lather. Rinse off with cool water.

17. ACTIVATED CHARCOAL SHAMPOO TO BOOST HAIR GROWTH

Ingredients:
- ¼ cup liquid Castile Soap (any variant)
- ¼ cup distilled water
- ½ teaspoon grapeseed or jojoba oil
- ¼ teaspoon activated charcoal
- Use a foaming bottle or flip-cap bottle for storage and dispensing

Procedure:

Mix all ingredients together (except the activated charcoal) and store in a dispenser. Shake well before use. To use, pour a tablespoon of the shampoo mixture into a bowl. Add a teaspoon of activated charcoal and mix well. Shampoo hair with the mixture. To boost hair growth, use this shampoo preparation once a week.

BATH BOMBS

Admit it. A bath bomb never fails to bring out the kid in you.   The fizz, the foam, and the bubbles always make your bathing experience such a joy.   The moisturizing oils give your skin a silky feel.   Right before your eyes, the water turns a pretty color; and the scent that gets released brings back happy memories.

So, wouldn't it be a blast if you could make your own personalized bath bombs?

MAKE YOUR OWN BATH BOMBS

Although bath bombs come in a wide variety of shapes, sizes, and colors, all bath bombs are made from the same base elements: baking soda, citric acid, and water. With a little change in each of the other components of a bath bomb, you'd be able to create your personalized recipes.

A combination of acid and base that's safe on your skin is what causes the fizz.   One part citric acid and two parts baking soda is a tried and tested ratio guaranteed to pack your bath bomb with tremendous fizz.   This acid-and-base combination should make up 60% of your dry ingredients.

The most commonly used fillers for bath bomb recipes are salts, grain powders, herb powders, honey powders, and clays. The more economical and readily available choice is cornstarch. Fillers make up the other 40% of the dry, powdered ingredients.

The two types of binding agents used in bath bomb recipes are oil and water. Whatever binding agent you choose, it should make up 10% to 20% of your entire recipe.

You may use either water-based or oil dispersible colorants. Remember that water-based dyes should be added to water-based binding agents or salts before incorporating them into the recipe. The same thing goes with oil dispersible colorants. They can only be added to oil-based binding agents. Be wary about using too much colorant as they may stain your skin and your bathroom fixtures.

You may use fragrance oils or essential oils for your aromatics. Your bath bomb recipe is not strict when it comes to the aromatics you wish to use as long as you keep in mind skin safety. A ratio of 1% to 5% of your total recipe should be enough. Leave your bath bombs unscented if your kids are likely to use them.

As additives, you may use dried petals, whole herbs, edible sprinkles, or sugar flowers. They may be embedded during molding or shaping.

Here are popular homemade bath bomb recipes.

1. BASIC BATH BOMB

Ingredients:
- ½ cup Epsom Salt
- 1 cup baking soda
- ½ cup corn starch
- ½ a cup citric acid
- 1 tablespoon water
- 1 tablespoon of your choice of essential oil
- 3 drops (1 teaspoon) fragrance
- Colorant

Procedure:
1. In a stainless steel bowl, blend all the dry ingredients together. Set aside.

2. In a glass jar with lid, mix all the wet ingredients until they

completely homogenize. Then whisk in the wet mixture bit by bit into dry mixture. Continue whisking until the mixture is the consistency of wet sand.

3. Scoop a portion of the mixture and press into a bath bomb mold. This recipe makes 4 baseball-sized bath bombs.

4. Air-dry your bath bombs for at least 3 hours before storing them in an airtight bag.

2. CHOCOLATE PEPPERMINT BATH BOMBS

Ingredients:
- ½ cup Epsom salt
- 1 cup baking soda
- ½ cup corn starch
- ½ cup citric acid
- 1 ounce cocoa butter
- ¼ cup buttermilk powder
- ¼ cup honey powder
- 1 ounce fractionated coconut oil
- 1 ounce vegetable glycerin
- 3 tablespoons cocoa powder
- 1 teaspoon peppermint oil
- 3 tablespoons parsley powder

Procedure:
1. Using a double boiler, melt cocoa butter. When melted, add in the glycerin and coconut oil, and then set aside.

2. In a large bowl, blend together Epsom salt and baking soda. Add the peppermint oil. Continue mixing. Add the citric acid, cornstarch, honey powder, buttermilk powder. Stir well.

3. Divide the mixture into two portions in separate bowls. Add in cocoa powder in the first portion, and parsley powder to the second portion.

4. Pour half of the cocoa butter mixture earlier set aside into the first bowl.   Knead the mixture with your hands. Then proceed molding individual bath bombs.

5. After you're done with the first bowl, add the remaining coco butter mixture to the other bowl, knead, and mold.

6. Let your bath bombs dry and harden, and then store them in an airtight container.

3. MILK AND HONEY BATH BOMBS

Ingredients:
- 3 tablespoons honey powder
- 3 tablespoons whole milk powder
- 2 cups baking soda
- 1 cup citric acid
- 3 tablespoons oatmeal
- 3 tablespoons chamomile flower powder
- 2 ounces witch hazel extract (pour in a sprayer bottle)
- 1 tablespoon of your favorite essential oil

Procedure:
1. In a big mixing bowl, mix the oil and baking soda.   Stir well to mix completely.

2. Add in the honey powder, whole milk powder, oatmeal, flower powder.

3. Add the citric acid. Continue mixing.

4. Wet the powder mixture with 10 spritz of the hazel witch, and then mix. Repeat until the mixture has the consistency of wet sand.

5. For the molds, you may use fancy shapes, such as star or heart-shaped molds.   Let the bath bombs dry and harden for 12 hours while in their molds.   Pack in an airtight container.

4. BATH FIZZIES

Ingredients:
- 1 cup baking soda
- 2 cups citric acid
- 1-1/2 ounces witch hazel hydrosol (combine with ½ ounce alcohol in a spray bottle)
- Colorant of your choice
- ½ teaspoon essential oil
- ½ ounce alcohol

Procedure:

1. In a mixing bowl, put together the powdered ingredients. Add the colorant and the essential oil. Mix well.

2. Wet the powder mixture with 10 sprays of the witch hazel-alcohol mixture, the stir immediately until the mixture is moist enough for molding.

3. Pack the mixture tightly into molds and leave to dry for 4 hours. Once your fizzies have completely hardened, remove them from the molds and pack in foils or airtight plastic containers.

5. COCO-LIME BATH COOKIES

Ingredients:
- 1 cup cornstarch
- ½ cup citric acid
- 1 cup baking soda
- ¾ cup brown sugar
- 1 tablespoon cocoa powder
- 1 cup rice bran powder
- 1 cup coconut milk powder, divided for mixture and for topping
- 2 ounces virgin coconut cream oil
- 5 teaspoons lime essential oil
- 2 ounces mango butter

Procedure:

1. Using a double boiler, warm and melt coconut cream oil and mango butter.   Set aside.

2. In a mixing bowl, combine cornstarch, cocoa powder, rice bran powder, brown sugar, and coconut milk powder. Mix thoroughly making sure that lumps don't form.

3. In another mixing bowl, combine citric acid and baking soda. Stir well, and then add in the mixture into the first bowl. Mix some more.

4. Pour the lime essential oil to the coconut-oil-mango-butter melted mixture, and then pour the liquid into the dry ingredients.

5. Knead the mixture thoroughly.   Form tablespoon-sized balls using your hands.   Roll the balls in coconut milk powder, coating them completely. Place the balls in a baking sheet lined with wax paper and flatten them with your palm until they are the shape of gingersnaps. Let the cookies dry for 24 hours.   Afterwards, you may pack them in ziplock bags.

6. RAINBOW-SPRINKLED BATH COOKIES

Ingredients:
- 1 cup cornstarch
- 1 cup baking soda
- ½ cup oatmeal
- ½ cup citric acid
- ¾ cup Epsom salt
- 2 ounces mango butter
- ¼ cup honey granules
- ¼ cup whole milk powder
- 2 ounces virgin coconut oil
- ½ teaspoon edible sprinkle

Procedure:

1. In a mixing bowl, blend together Epsom salt, cornstarch, oatmeal, and whole milk powder. Break up clumps that may form. Add in the honey granules.

2. In a double boiler, melt the virgin coconut cream oil and mango butter.

3. In another bowl, mix together citric acid and baking soda. Pour in the melted oil mixture while stirring constantly. Continue kneading the mixture with your hands.

4. Form small balls. Arrange them in a baking sheet lined with wax paper. Press each ball with your palms to flatten them into cookie shapes. Place sprinkles on top and press some more. Let the cookies dry overnight in a cool and dry place. Store your cookies in a sealed container.

7. WHOOPIE BATH TUB PIES

Part 1: Making the Chocolate Cookies

Dry Ingredients:
- 1 cup baking soda
- ¾ cup Epsom salt
- ½ cup citric acid
- ½ cup fine oat flour
- ½ cup whole milk powder
- 1 teaspoon umber oxide
- ½ cup cocoa powder

Wet Ingredients:
- Fragrance oil
- ½ ounce dark chocolate supreme
- 2 ounces cocoa butter
- 1 ounce virgin coconut oil

Procedure:

1. In a mixing bowl, stir all the dry ingredients together. Break up any clumps that may form. You may opt to mix the dry ingredients in a blender or food processor.

2. Using a double boiler, melt cocoa butter.

3. Combine the wet ingredients in a bowl. Pour in the melted cocoa butter and stir well.

4. Gradually pour the liquid ingredients into the bowl of dry powders. Stir the mixture vigorously making sure that mixture is the consistency of wet sand and is moist for shaping. This is your Whoopie pie mixture. Make small balls with your hands, and then further divide each ball into halves to make cookie pairs. Arrange the cookie pairs in a baking sheet lined with wax paper. Press each piece such that they take the shape of small mounds.

5. Allow your cookies to dry for 48 hours or longer for as long as they sit in some cool, dry place.

Part 2: The Icing

Ingredients:
- 1 teaspoon butter cream fragrance oil
- 2 teaspoons beeswax
- 1 teaspoon cornstarch
- 1 teaspoon white kaolin clay
- 1 cup shealoe butter

Procedure:

1. Melt beeswax using a double boiler. Once melted, remove from flame and throw in the shealoe butter. Stir the mixture constantly. Add in the kaolin clay and cornstarch into the double boiler while continuously whipping the mixture until it cools.

2. When the mixture in the double boiler is already thoroughly mixed, pour it into a mixing bowl. Whisk the mixture until it cools to room temperature.

3. Add in the butter cream fragrance oil. Continue whisking.

4. Transfer the mixture into a pastry bag. Make sure though that the bag's tip is still sealed. Set aside in a cool, dry place for the next part of the preparation.

Part 3: Assembling your Whoopies

After 48 hours, the cookies must have set already and have hardened up enough to pick up without crumbling. If the icing was prepared on the same day the cookies were made, then it must have hardened just as well. Apply frosting tip to the pastry bag. You will be frosting one cookie from each pair. The other is one is for sandwiching.

Begin frosting from the center of the cookie and spiral out towards the edges. Then top with its pair. Let the complete whoopies sit for a couple of days more to harden. Keep them moist-free in an airtight jar.

BATH SALTS

Bath salts are water-soluble minerals used to add health benefits water to be used for bathing. These salts serve as bases for cleaning and cosmetic agents. Bath salts are often used as an alternative to natural thermal baths or springs. The most common ingredient in bath salts is glycerine which is very important in keeping your skin lubricated, hydrated, and moisturized.

Bath salts can sometimes be sold as Epsom salt, table salt, baking soda, and borax.

BENEFITS OF BATH SALTS

- The naturally-occurring minerals and nutrients in pure bath salts help keep your skin supple and radiant. These minerals include potassium (checks the balance of moisture levels in skin), magnesium (fights stress and combats fatigue), bromide (sooths sore muscles), calcium (promotes strong bones), and sodium (manages the balance of lymphatic fluids). They are easily absorbed through skin pores and therefore benefit not only your skin but your whole body from the inside out.
- Using bath salts in your warm bath helps draw out dirt and pollution from your skin.
- Bath salts are known to help manage the discomfort brought about by tendinitis and osteoarthritis.
- Bath salts also provide relief from itchiness, psoriasis, and insomnia.
- As a result of all the foregoing, you look younger because you feel rejuvenated, calm, and generally happy.
- If you bathe in the morning, bath salts together with your favorite essential oil will perk you up and get you to start your day highly-energized.

MAKING YOUR OWN BATH SALTS

The setup and procedure across the many bath salt recipes are somewhat similar. Here are a few variations that you can try.

1. GREEN TEA AND PEPPERMINT BATH SALTS

Ingredients:
- 1 cup sea salt, finely-ground
- 3 cups Epsom salt
- 4 drops peppermint essential oil
- 9 green tea bags
- 6 drops fractionated coconut oil if you have dry skin (or almond oil if you have oily skin)

Procedure:

1. In a medium-sized bowl, combine sea salt and Epsom salt. Stir well.

2. Cut open the green tea bags and add the contents to the salt mixture. Stir some more.

3. Add the peppermint oil, the coconut or almond oil, and mix well. Cover the mixing bowl with a tower and set aside for an hour.

4. Transfer your bath salt in an airtight container and store in a dry place.

2. BUBBLING BATH SALTS

Ingredients:
- 1/3 cup body wash (unscented)
- 2 cups Epsom salt
- 2 drops lavender essential oil
- 1 teaspoon jojoba oil
- 2 drops food coloring

Procedure:

1. Place the Epsom in a bowl. Add in the body wash, the jojoba oil, the lavender essential oil, and the colorant.   Stir well.

2. Spread the salt mixture on cookie sheet and leave to dry for 24 hours. Stir every so often to dry evenly and make sure that you break up any chunks and the mixture doesn't stick together.

3. Transfer your bath salt in a mason jar.   To use, add ¼ cup of this bath salt to your tub before you get in.

3. DETOX BATH SALTS

Ingredients:
- 1 cup Epsom salt
- 5 drops citrus essential oil
- 5 drops lavender essential oil
- Lavender flowers

Procedure:

1. In a stainless steel bowl, mix together the Epsom and the essential oils. Mix together well with a metal spoon.

2. Transfer your mixture in a mason jar. Put a spoonful of lavender flowers on top and seal.

3. To use, add 2 tablespoons of salt in your tub.

4. BEDTIME BATH SALTS

Ingredients:
- Epsom salt
- Sweet almond essential oil
- Vitamin E oil
- 10 drops valor essential oil
- 15 drops RC essential oil
- 15 drops lavender essential oil
- Extra coarse bath salt

Procedure:

1. Fill a container with Epsom salt up to an inch off the lid. Fill the remaining inch with the extra coarse bath salts.

2. Pour the proportioned salts mixture in a glass bowl and stir well.

3. Add in the almond oil. Mix well as the mixture will turn clumpy.

4. Add in the oils including vitamin E oil. Continue mixing.

5. Pour the mixture into a mason jar and seal.

6. To use, put ¼ cup in your tub.

5. BATH SALTS FOR BACK PAIN

Ingredients:
- 1 cup baking soda
- 2 cups Epsom salts
- 5 drops cinnamon essential oil
- 5 drops lavender essential oil
- 5 drops rosemary essential oil
- 5 drops eucalyptus essential oil
- 10 drops peppermint essential oil
- 1 tablespoon fresh rosemary springs
- 2 tablespoons dried lavender flowers

Procedure:

1. Mix Epsom salts and baking soda in a large bowl.   Add in all the essential oils. Stir well to distribute the oils evenly.

2. Stir in the rosemary springs and lavender flowers.

3. Transfer salts in a jar and store in a dry place.

4. To use, put 1 cup of bath salts in your tub.

6. DECONGESTANT BATH SALTS

Ingredients:
- ½ cup baking soda
- 1 cup Epsom salt
- 10 drops eucalyptus essential oils
- 5 drops peppermint essential oils
- Green food color

Procedure:

1. Mix together the baking soda and Epsom salts. Add in the colorant.   Stir well until the salts are an even color.

2. Add in the eucalyptus and peppermint oils. Mix together well and then transfer in a jar.

3. To use, put a few scoops in your warm water.

BODY SCRUBS

Exfoliate, clarify and hydrate! Here are easy-to-make body scrubs recipes. Because of the organic ingredients that may spoil easily, it is recommended that you prepare only a batch for each single use.

1. BANANA SUGAR BODY SCRUB

Ingredients:
- 3 tablespoons granulated sugar
- 1 ripe banana
- ¼ teaspoon of your favorite essential oil

Procedure:

1. Mash the banana with a fork. Set aside some banana for use in your face.

2. Add granulated sugar and oil into the banana into a goop.

3. To use, pat the banana-sugar mixture and massage all over your body.

4. Use the plain banana you set aside to massage your face except the eyes.

5. Rinse off with warm water.

2. STARTER SUGAR SCRUB

Ingredients:
- 1 part olive oil
- 3 parts sugar
- 15 drops of your favorite essential oil

Procedure:

1. Combine all the ingredients in a mason jar. Stir well.

2. To use, scoop a generous amount and massage on your knees, elbows, feet, and everywhere else you need it.

3. CITRUS SALT SCRUB

Ingredients:
- 1 teaspoon citrus zest (grapefruit, lemon, lime, or orange)
- ½ cup sea salt
- ½ cup essential oil of your choice

Procedure:

1. Mix all the ingredients together and store in a jar.

2. To use, rub on skin (avoiding the eyes) while in the shower.

3. Rinse off.

4. COCONUT-VANILLA BROWN SUGAR SCRUB

Ingredients:
- ½ teaspoon vanilla
- ½ cup coconut oil
- ½ cup brown sugar

Procedure:

1. Mix all the ingredients together.

2. Rub on skin while in the shower.

3. Massage thoroughly.

4. Rinse off.

5. COCONUT-OATMEAL SCRUB

Ingredients:
- 1 teaspoon brown sugar
- 1 teaspoon honey
- 1 teaspoon vanilla extract
- ½ cup organic coconut oil
- 1-1/2 cups oatmeal

Procedure:

1. Grind oatmeal using a food processor. Transfer into a bowl.

2. Add brown sugar into the oatmeal and mix well.

3. Put in honey, coconut oil, and vanilla into the oatmeal mixture. Mix well.

4. Store in an airtight container.

5. Use as how you would body scrubs.

6. GINGER SUGAR FACE AND BODY SCRUB

Ingredients:
- ¼ cup kosher salt
- ¾ cup granulated sugar
- ¼ cup of your favorite essential oil
- 1 tablespoon coarsely chopped ginger
- ¼ cup coconut oil
- 4 drops lemongrass essential oil

Procedure:

1. In a saucepan, heat the ginger and coconut oil for 5-10 minutes until the ginger juice and scent get into the oil. Remove from heat and filter oil into a glass container.

2. Mix in your choice of essential oil. Stir well to combine and let the mixture cool down to room temperature.

3. Stir in salt and sugar. Add lemongrass oil.

4. To use, rub on face and let stay for 2 minutes. Wet a face towel with warm water and place on your face. Then wipe off and rinse off oils.

5. Do the same with the rest of your body.

7. HONEY AND BLUEBERRY SCRUB

Ingredients:
- 1 teaspoon fine sugar
- 1/3 cup fresh blueberries
- 2 tablespoons honey
- ½ teaspoon green tea

Procedure:

1. Mash the blueberries with a fork.

2. Mix together blueberries, green tea, honey and sugar in a container.   Stir well.

3. To use, apply a generous layer on your skin.   Leave it there for 15 minutes.

4. Rinse off with lukewarm water while doing circular motions.

8. VANILLA ROSE SUGAR SCRUB RECIPE

Ingredients:
- 2 small roses, chopped
- 1 teaspoon Vitamin E oil
- 1 vanilla bean
- 10 drops rose essential oil
- ¾ cup sweet almond oil
- 1 cup granulated sugar

Procedure:

1. Blend together sugar, almond oil, rose oil, and vitamin E.

2. Remove the seeds from your vanilla bean. Mix the seeds with your scrub.

3. Mix in the rose petals. Mix some more.

4. Use as how you would other body scrubs.

BODY LOTION / MOISTURIZER

1. BASIC HOMEMADE LOTION

Ingredients:
- ¼ cup beeswax
- ¼ cup coconut oil
- ½ cup jojoba oil
- 1 teaspoon Vitamin E oil

Procedure:

1. Combine and melt beeswax, coconut oil, and jojoba oil in a double boiler.   Mix thoroughly.

2. When completely melted, add the vitamin E oil. Mix some more.

3. Pour the mixture in a jar.   This mixture is quite thick for storage in a lotion pump.

4. Use like you would a regular lotion for ultra-moisturizing effect. This recipe is also great for diaper rash and stretch marks.

5. Shelf life is 6 months.

2. ALOE-BASED LOTION

Ingredients:
- 1 cup aloe vera gel
- ½ cup almond oil
- 1 teaspoon + 1 tablespoon beeswax
- 1 teaspoon vitamin E oil
- 10 drops geranium essential oil

Procedure:

1. Melt almond oil and beeswax in a double boiler. Remove from heat and mix using a stick blender.

2. Let the mixture cool to room temperature.   Then add the vitamin E and geranium essential oils.

3. Blend some with the stick blender set to low. Gradually add in the aloe vera gel until completely incorporated.

4. Store in a glass jar and keep inside the ref.

5. Discard unused lotion after 6 weeks.

3. REFRESHING ALOE-MINT LOTION

Ingredients:
- ½ cup aloe vera gel
- 1/8 teaspoon peppermint essential oil
- 1 cup coconut oil
- ¼ cup beeswax

Procedure:

1. Melt the coconut oil and beeswax in a double boiler over low heat.

2. Remove the melted mixture from the heat.   Immediately pour in peppermint essential oil and aloe vera gel.   Stir well.

3. Let the lotion cool down to room temperature, and then whisk to make it fluffy.

4. Over time, some of the aloe juice will evaporate and the lotion will naturally turn thicker.

4. LOTION FOR ECZEMA

Ingredients:
- ¼ cup coconut oil
- 5 drops tea tree essential oil
- 15 drops lavender essential oil
- ¼ cup shea butter

Procedure:

1. Using a double boiler, melt the coconut oil and shea butter. Let cool to room temperature.

2. Add in the essential oils and fluff the mixture using a stick blender.

3. Transfer the mixture in a mason jar.   Store in the ref.

4. To use, apply liberally on the affected skin.

5. NON-GREASY SUMMER LOTION

Ingredients:
- ½ cup aloe vera gel
- ½ cup distilled water
- ¼ cup jojoba oil
- ¼ cup fractionated coconut oil
- ½ cup beeswax pastilles
- 16 drops essential oil of your choice
- 1 teaspoon Vitamin E

Procedure:

1. Combine aloe vera gel and water in a bowl.

2. Melt the beeswax in a double boiler over medium.   Let cool a little then add the essential oils.   Blend together well.

3. Bring the water temperature within the same temperature as the beeswax.

4. Put the aloe-water and beeswax mixtures and the vitamin E oil in a blender and blend for 15 minutes until fluffy.

5. Use like you would regular lotion.

6. Any leftovers past the 3 month mark should be discarded.

6. BASIC LOTION BAR

Ingredients:
- 1/3 cup beeswax pastilles
- 1/3 cup jojoba oil
- 1/3 cup fractionated coconut oil
- 8 drops essential oil of your choice

Procedure:

1. Melt beeswax and jojoba oil in a double boiler.

2. Remove from heat and mix in the essential oils. Pour into molds. Let cool.

3. To use, rub your bar until some of it melts into your hands. Proceed to apply it on your skin.

7. THE 2000-YEAR-OLD LOTION RECIPE

Ingredients:
- 7 ounces almond oil
- 8 tablespoons beeswax pastille
- 1 tablespoon raw honey
- ½ cup rosewater

Procedure:

1. Melt the almond oil, beeswax, and raw honey in a double boiler over low heat. Then remove from heat and allow to cool slight.

2. Add in the rosewater gradually until fully blended.

3. Pour the mixture in a clean jar and let cool before covering.

4. Keep refrigerated.

8. ORANGE HONEY LOTION BARS

Ingredients:
- 2 ounces olive oil
- 2 ounces coconut oil
- ounces shea butter
- 2 ounces ounces beeswax
- 1-½ tablespoons raw honey
- 6 drops orange essential oil

Procedure:

1. In a double boiler, melt the coconut oil, shea butter, beeswax. Mix well.

2. Turn the flame off and add orange essential oils, olive oil, and honey

3. Pour into molds. You may use muffin tins with cup cake liners.

4. Allow the mixture to harden within 8 hours. You may put them in the ref to expedite the process.

5. To use, rub your bar until some of it melts into your hands. Proceed to apply it on your skin.

9. SUNSCREEN LOTION BAR

Ingredients:
- 2 tablespoons zinc oxide
- ½ teaspoon Vitamin E oil
- ½ cup coconut oil
- 5 tablespoons beeswax
- ½ cup shea butter
- ¾ teaspoon lavender essential oil (avoid citrus oils as they induce photosensitivity)

Procedure:

1. Melt the beeswax, shea butter, and coconut oil on low in a double boiler on low flame.   Stir well until fully incorporated.

2. Remove from heat. Add in the zinc oxide, vitamin E oil, and essential oil.

3. Pour into a silicone mold and let cool for about 30 minutes in the refrigerator.

4. Unmold and store in an airtight container at room temperature.

5. To use, rub your bar until some of it melts into your hands. Proceed to apply it on your skin.

10. SKIN-SOOTHING LOTION

Ingredients:
- 1 ounce emulsifying wax (do not substitute beeswax)
- 2 tablespoons citric acid (or use freshly-squeezed lemon juice)
- 2 tablespoons oatmeal
- ½ cup water
- ½ cup milk
- 1 ounce cocoa butter
- ¼ cup milk
- 1/3 cup almond oil

Procedure:

1. Pour oatmeal (that's been soaked in water overnight) in a processor.   Blend at high setting until smooth.

2. Slightly heat milk in a pan while being careful not to bring it to a boil. Remove from heat and transfer into a glass jar. Add in water.

3. In a double broiler, melt the emulsifying wax, cocoa butter, and almond oil while stirring constantly.   Remove from heat as as completely melted.

4. Pour the melted mixture into your jar of milk, stirring continuously until completely homogenized.

5. Add in the lemon juice and oatmeal. Stir with a clean spoon. Let cool for an hour.   Stir the mixture at intervals of 10 minutes.

6. Place in the refrigerator after every use.

7. Apply on your skin and let stay for a while before taking a shower or bath.

8. Remember that because this recipe contains organic ingredients, it has the tendency to spoil due to unsanitary handling.   Use a clean stick (not your fingers) to scoop a portion for every use.

BODY BUTTERS

Body butter is a skin moisturizer that could be used as substitute for lotion. It's generally made with skincare butters like cocoa butter, shea butter, and mango butter.

1. LUXURIOUS WHIPPED BODY BUTTER

Ingredients:
- ½ cup almond oil
- ½ cup coconut oil
- ½ cup mango butter
- ½ cup shea butter
- 30 drops lavender essential oil

Procedures:
1. Melt all the ingredients in a double boiler set on medium flame. Remove and allow to cool slightly. Add in the lavender oil.

2. Put the mixture in the refrigerator for an hour to harden a little.

3. Using a hand mixer, whip the mixture for 10 minutes until fluffy.

4. Put back the mixture in the refrigerator and leave it for 10 minutes to set.

5. Transfer into a glass jar with lid.

6. Use as how you would regular body butter or lotion.

2. NOURISHING & MOISTURIZING BODY BUTTER

Ingredients:
- ¼ cup carrier oil
- ¼ cup cocoa butter
- ¼ cup shea butter
- 36 drops essential oil

Procedure:

1. Melt the butters in a double boiler.   Remove from heat as soon as fully melted.

2. Add in the carrier oil and stir well.   Allow to cool down, and then place in the refrigerator to harden.

3. When the mixture turns opaque and a little hard, remove from the refrigerator.   Add in the essential oil.

4. Whisk the mixture using a fork until it's visibly whipped.

5. Transfer into a jar with lid. Store at room temperature.

6. To use, scoop a small amount using your fingertips and then apply on your skin.

3.   SHEA & LAVENDER BODY BUTTER

Ingredients:
- 1/8 cup sweet almond oil
- 1/8 cup coconut oil
- ¼ cup shea butter, unrefined
- 10 drops lavender essential oil

Procedure:

1. Melt coconut oil and butter in a double boiler over medium flame. Remove from heat as soon as fully melted.   Let cool a little.

2. Add in the sweet almond oil and lavender oil. Stir well.

3. Transfer the mixture into a glass bowl.

4. Chill the mixture in the freezer for 10 minutes. Allow to harden a little.

5. Using a hand mixer, whip the mixture and then transfer in an airtight container.

6. Use as how you would regular lotion.

4. ORANGE & COCONUT BODY BUTTER

Ingredients:
- 2 drops sweet almond oil
- 1-1/2 tablespoons shea butter
- ½ cup coconut oil
- 25 drops orange essential oil

Procedure:

1. Bring together almond oil, shea butter, and coconut oil in a medium bowl.

2. Using a hand mixer, blend the ingredients together. Add in the essential oil and mix some more for 5 minutes until the mixture turns fluffy.

3. Transfer the mixture into a glass container with a lid. Refrigerate if needed.

FACE MASKS

1. THE HYDRATING AVOCADO MASK

Ingredients and Procedure:

1. Mash ½ an avocado with a fork. Add in a teaspoon of honey and a teaspoon of yogurt and continue mixing into a paste.

2. Apply on your clean face and leave it on for 15 minutes.

3. Rinse off with lukewarm water.

2. COCOA HYDRATION MASK

Ingredients and Procedure:

1. Get a quarter of avocado and mash in a small bowl.

2. Add in 1 tablespoon honey and 1 tablespoon cocoa powder. Mash and mix some more.

3. Clean your face and dry up. Apply the mask and leave it on for 10 minutes.

4. Rinse off with lukewarm water.

5. Moisturize.

3. THE BREAKFAST MASK

Ingredients and Procedure:

1. Put together 1 egg yolk, 1 tablespoon of olive oil, 1 tablespoon of honey, and half a cup of oatmeal. Stir well.

2. Apply on your clean face and leave it on for 15-20 minutes.

3. Rinse with lukewarm water.

4. Moisturize.

4. PAPAYA LIGHTENING MASK

Ingredients and Procedure:

1. Mix together half a cup of mashed papaya and 2 tablespoons of honey.

2. Apply gently on your clean face and leave it on for 20 minutes.

3. Wash off.

4. Moisturize.

5. HONEY CITRUS MASK

Ingredients and Procedure:

1. Mix 3 tablespoons orange juice with ¼ cup honey.

2. Gently rub over your face. Leave it on for 15 minutes.

3. Rinse off with lukewarm water.

4. Moisturize.

Excited to try these out? Well, before you do, here are a few more things to keep in mind:

- Check for any allergies you might have. Sure, the ingredients for many of these recipes are organic and safe for use in most cases, but do be careful if you're aware of any food related allergies that you have. It's best to do a skin patch test before trying anything out.

- Always wear safety gear. This is especially so if you're handing ingredients for soap making. Prepare everything beforehand and make sure to stow them away from the equipment you use for making other bath products.

So there you have it! We hope the information provided here and the recipes that go along with it help in boosting your bath time experience. Best of all, you can even turn this into a small business or simply something you can make for family and friends once you really get the hang of it.

We wish you the best of luck!